Very Common NonAlcoholic Fatty Liver Disease

How To Know if You Have Hepatic Steatosis

By: James M. Lowrance © 2013

TABLE OF CONTENTS:

INTRODUCTION:

(This eBook is approximately 3,120 words in length.)

Most of the general population is not well informed about a common condition affecting the liver, that affects an estimated 29 million people in America alone. Up to 6.5 million of these people, will go on to experience inflammation in their livers or what is also referred to as "steatohepatitis".

Many will eventually experience cirrhosis in their livers, meaning scarring/lesions that will begin to appear within the organ, which is irreversible and that can eventually lead to death or in the need for a life-saving liver transplant.

The author whose words you are reading in this book/ebook, is a patient who has lived with a condition of non-alcoholic fatty liver, since the year 2007 (for six years at the time of this writing).

4

My case of the disease has not gone on to become steatohepatitis but I have been diagnosed with enlargement of my liver, which is reversible at this point, if I follow my doctor's treatments and a weight loss plan (my obesity is between moderate and severe). While I am not a medical professional, I am one who can relate facts concerning this disease, from firsthand experience with it. I can also pass along the knowledge I have accrued, through six years of extensive research on literally hundreds of reputable medical websites, as well as from blogs and articles written by fellow liver disease patients. While the information I will relate is not as extensive as that one could contain through a professional medical journal, I do believe I can express information that most laypersons would be seeking, in addition to sharing my personal experience with this potentially very serious disease.

It is my sincere hope that the information which follows within the succeeding chapters, will prove to be beneficial to the readers who obtain it.

CHAPTER ONE:

What is Non-Alcoholic Fatty Liver Disease (NAFLD)?

This condition that largely affects adults, is also affecting an alarming number of children as well and is strongly associated with obesity and lack of physical activity (exercise).

When obesity is chronic – lasting for years, the liver will begin to store larger amounts of fat over time, until a large portion of its cells are comprised of fat, rather than being comprised of natural liver cells. The liver is the body's largest organ and it plays a major role in body-fat metabolism, which is called "gluconeogenesis".

The liver also plays a major role in synthesizing (balancing) and metabolizing (creating energy for the body) via the management of other essential substances, such as sugar, cholesterol and triglycerides.

The organ manages bodily metabolism, by converting carbohydrates from foods that are consumed, into glucose to be used in all cells of the body, for energy to operate adequately. Glucose (metabolized sugar), is an essential hormone, that provides fuel for organs in the body to operate properly, including the brain and they are highly dependent upon this daily fuel, that it provides.

When looking at carbohydrates coming into the body, the term "calories", may be used, which is basically a measurement of how many units are needed to maintain healthy levels of energy and how too many units/calories, can be stored in the body, rather than being burned-up as energy, as the body operates to fulfill daily tasks. Depending on the age, sex and activities of an individual, the number of calories needed per day, can range anywhere from 1,000 to 2,800 per day. When all of these factors are considered and a person exceeds their calorie needs, the liver will instead convert carbohydrates into fat and store it for future needs.

This would be similar to how some animals store fat as they go into winter-time hibernation, so that their bodies survive extended periods of inactivity, during which they also do not consume any carbohydrates. However, people do not hibernate in the true sense, as some animals do and as they gain/store fat in their bodies, which also shows outwardly, in addition to increasing inwardly, they do not stop the excessive calorie trend. Their abnormally high fat accumulation, is carried through each season of the year and may continue to build each year as well (chronic weight gain).

Humans are different from the hibernating animals previously mentioned, and hibernation is not a necessary mechanism that is built into us. We rather continue our activities ear-round, although those activities may change in intensity at certain times of the year. For those who live in areas of the world where there is a strong contrast between winter and summer months – with winter usually being a time of less activity, less calories are usually needed but may not be reduced accordingly.

For most people, calorie-counting is not a necessary practice because we have a built-in hunger mechanism that tells us when we need to consume more calories or less of them.

For people who abuse their diets however, this hunger mechanism will change negatively and cravings for unnecessarily larger amounts of calories and for foods that are very high in refined sugars will begin to occur (e.g. cravings for candies, cakes, cookies, pies and soft drinks will increase).

Cravings for foods that are normally healthy in proper moderation, will also become increasingly craved, such as those containing natural, but high glucose content such as potatoes, white rice, corn,dairy products and breads (pastas are also bread products).

Unfortunately the industrial food manufacturing world, has evolved into many businesses who have continued to expand their lines of junk foods and high sugar-content soft drinks.

As a result, this trend has contributed to a number of metabolic problems within the world community, including obesity, diabetes, metabolic syndrome (pre-diabetes – insulin resistance) and **non-alcoholic fatty liver disease.**

CHAPTER TWO:

What Are the Symptoms and Methods for Diagnosing NAFLD?

NAFLD, usually presents with no noticeable symptoms. However, when the condition becomes severe enough and fatty infiltration has developed throughout the liver, symptoms may begin to manifest. Those that can become most prominent, are fatigue, flu-like symptoms and a feeling of fullness or vague pain occurring on the right side of the abdomen, extending upward into the ribcage. This is the area where the approximately 3.5 lb organ is located but when swelling occurs, pain and feelings of being bloated, may become evident.

For most people with NAFLD, symptoms do not occur and they do not become aware of the condition, until it reaches a severity that results in inflammation or what is also referred to as "hepatitis"(more on fatty liver hepatitis will be discussed in the next chapter).

NAFLD usually is found incidentally, when a person has gone to their doctor for a checkup and blood testing is ordered, to include a "metabolic panel". This set of blood tests, will include a measure of "liver enzymes", which are cells produced by the liver and that are released into the bloodstream at higher than normal elevations, when damage to the organ is occurring.

Damage that causes elevations in these liver enzymes, the main ones being the "ALT" and the "AST", can result from a number of different types of hepatitis, many of which do not involve fatty liver conditions but that result from certain types of viral infections and drug or alcohol abuse.

Hepatitis viruses include the A, B, C, D, and G types, with the **A, B, and C** being the most common infections. When a patient's blood test shows elevations of liver enzymes, their doctor will usually opt to test them for these types of viruses, via a "hepatitis panel".

This step would simply be one of precaution, especially if viral hepatitis symptoms are not occurring, such as jaundice (yellowing of the skin), joint pain and itching, and if a patient is not an intravenous drug user and does not engage in promiscuous sex (common ways to contract the viral types of hepatitis).

Once it is established that elevations in liver enzymes are not the result of viral hepatitis illnesses, a treating doctor can then attribute the blood abnormalities to non-alcoholic fatty liver disease. A common sign that reveals NAFLD as being the type present, would be obesity and less-commonly, a patient who simply consumes excessive amounts of fatty foods in their diets, but who has not become obviously obese.

A doctor would then refer the patient for a more definitive test, called a "liver ultrasound", which is a highly detailed look at the organ, through the use if sound waves that are sent toward all areas of liver tissue.

This test will determine if fatty cell infiltration has occurred and how far along the condition has progressed. A measurement of the organ would also be taken, to see if enlargement has occurred as well.

This test is the same type that is used to view the unborn fetuses if pregnant women and that is so detailed, that it can actually determine the fetus' sex and physical development. When the test is directed at a patient's liver, the surface of the organ will have a slick, shiny appearance, if fatty infiltration has occurred.

CHAPTER THREE:

When Does NAFLD Become Non-Alcoholic SteatoHepatitis (NASH) and How is It Treated?

In some cases of NAFLD, inflammation will begin to occur, even if a patient is unaware of it because hepatitis symptoms have yet to occur. Once inflammation has set in, the condition is then referred to as "Non-Alcoholic Steatohepatitis" ("NASH"). If an ultrasound of the organ, shows a fatty infiltration appearance, the ordering doctor may then refer the patient to a surgeon, who can perform a liver biopsy. With this test, a small tissue sample will be taken via a method called a "percutaneous biopsy". With this method, a hollow needle is inserted into the abdomen, to extract a small tissue sample from the liver and this may be done as an outpatient procedure or as a hospital surgery.

The sample is then analyzed to see if significant damage is occurring from fatty liver hepatitis.

In some cases, if the inflammatory disease has not begun to cause irreversible damage, a patient may be able to follow a treatment plan, that will save the organ from eventual death and failure. If NASH is diagnosed a treatment regimen would still be implemented, in attempt to slow progression of the disease, as much as possible and to attempt a reversal of it (a possibility at early stages).

Treatments that may be given to patients with NASH, would include weight loss, first and foremost, via a sensible diet plan and abstaining from alcohol (while alcohol is not the cause, it can be harmful to fatty liver conditions).

However, patients with the disease may also be given medications that are usually prescribed to diabetic patients such as insulin boosting drugs, like the major brand "Metformin" and drugs to help lower cholesterol, called "statin medications", including brands – Lipitor, Zocor, Mevacor, Pravachol or Crestor.

The treating doctor must observe a patient's response to these drugs with repeat blood testing. While the goal of them is to lower cholesterol, the medications can rarely in some cases, actually worsen liver disease (rare). This is why repeat blood testing of liver enzyme levels, becomes necessary as well, to see if they are decreasing or increasing.

Fatty liver diseases of both NAFLD and NASH, result from conditions called "Metabolic Syndromes" and these are referred to as such because they adversely affect the metabolism of individuals who have developed them.

The metabolic effects include imbalances in cholesterol and glucose (sugar) levels, which can also affect blood pressure, causing hypertension. This also places these patients at risk for developing diabetes because metabolic syndromes are also considered pre-diabetic illnesses.

When diabetes also develops in NAFLD and NASH patients, the diabetes must be aggressively treated because the combination of them presents a greater challenge to both doctor and patient, to prevent a more serious progression of the liver disease.

If NASH fails to be treated adequately via patient cooperation with diet changes and a lifestyle of regular exercise, liver failure can eventually develop. This can mean eventual death for the patient or in them requiring a liver transplant, to save their lives and to extend the number of years in their lifespan. Many patients with NASH, do not experience serious illness or eventual liver failure but a significant number of them do. This is the reason why it is so important for NAFLD patients to adhere faithfully to treatment plans that can reverse their fatty live conditions and to prevent the development of NASH.

CHAPTER FOUR:

My Own NAFLD Story

In the year 2007, I went to my doctor for a checkup and part of this follow up visit, was to recheck my thyroid hormone levels, with my being a treated hypothyroid patient (underactive thyroid gland). My doctor ordered me a "thyroid panel" but he also ordered me a "Complete Blood Count" (CBC) and a metabolic panel. Additionally, he ordered a "Hemoglobin A1C", which is a test that shows the average glucose levels of the person being tested, for a 2 to 3 month period. My results all came back normal, except for my ALT and AST liver enzyme levels, both of which were moderately elevated. I knew immediately that this was not good and I discussed with my doctor, what the meaning of these abnormal test results were.

He explained to me that my moderate obesity (at that time), was causing an accumulation of fat cells in my liver.

He explained that these fat cells caused normal liver tissue to become damaged and to release the ALT and AST enzymes into the bloodstream. My elevations were not terribly high but only 30 or 40 points above the normal values range for each. My doctor informed me that weight loss could lower the abnormally high liver blood counts and that eating a diet with plenty of fiber included, could also help to reduce build-up of fat cells. I was not prescribed any medications at that point but my doctor was firm in warning me to avoiding a worsening liver problem, through continued weight loss and by following a routine of sustained exercise.

As I would be retested on my liver blood counts each year, they would fluctuate from being 50 points above normal, to only 10 points above normal. My body weight was not fluctuating but was actually increasing yearly. Part of this was due to aging, which usually slows down activities in older people and part of it was my bad diet practices, that I still had not corrected. I was still consuming refined sugars in junk foods on a regular basis.

I was however also eating healthy foods, which in my mind, would offset the bad part of my diet (largely not true). I was also getting a fairly regular load of exercise with my work duties, which required heavy lifting at least twice weekly. I wasn't however, getting an adequate amount of sustained exercise, like one would get with regular walking or jogging and that my doctor strongly recommended. I was maintaining some of my muscle content but I was not getting adequate cardiovascular workouts.

With my continuing to consume fats and refined sugars and not getting proper exercise, my weight gain increased dramatically, during one particular years time. This was also due to a medication I was prescribed, to control my peripheral neuropathy symptoms (Gabapentin – for nerve pain in feet and legs), which developed before I was later diagnosed with diabetes. Peripheral neuropathy can result from metabolic syndromes and it does not have to be associated with diabetes.

In fact, approximately one-third pf peripheral neuropathy cases, have no causes found for them (idiopathic – no cause determined). After my year of increased weight gain, my blood was tested and my ALT and AST liver enzyme levels, were more that twice the highest normal cut off range! I knew this had reached a very serious point and placed me at risk for developing NASH.

My doctor sent me for a new liver ultrasound because of the very high elevations of liver enzymes. The report from the test came back negative for any scaring in my liver (cirrhosis) and it was negative for the presence of any tumors. The test did however, show that my liver had become somewhat enlarged to due the increased infiltration of fat cells. I am currently being treated for diabetes, with medications that can also contribute to reversing my fatty liver disease. At the time of this writing, I have lost approximately 15 lb of weight and I will continue to lose more, as I faithfully adhere to my low-fat, low-glucose diet.

I am also treated with a hypertensive medication for high blood pressure and a statin medication for a mildly elevated cholesterol level.

I would warn readers who have obtained this resource, to realize how potentially serious fatty liver disease can become. It has the potential to cause life-threatening cirrhosis, that is as severe as that found in people suffering from chronic alcoholism. Junk food addiction and addiction to rich, fatty foods, can be as difficult to break as an addiction to alcohol but neglecting to break those addictions, can have dire consequences when fatty liver disease is present.

I would recommend to those fatty liver disease patients, who have severe addictions to harmful foods, to seriously consider joining structured, reputable weight loss programs like "Weight Watchers" or "Jenny Craig" and to develop a regular exercise regimen (walking at least 1 hour weekly, is often preferred). These endeavors are somewhat difficult and take a fair degree of discipline to accomplish.

They are however, a far better trade against developing hepatitis that can be irreversible, ending in failure of life-supporting liver function and in being placed on a waiting list to receive a liver transplant.

I do hope that I have offered the preceding information within proper balance and that my warnings to fatty liver patients do not come across as sensationalistic scare tactics. The facts I have presented are true and being offered by me -- a non-medical layperson who has lived with a fatty liver condition since year-2007. I understand firsthand, the fears and struggles, this metabolic syndrome can bring. I also hope my shared information serves to inspire fellow fatty liver patients to take the initiative for living a full quality of life, as they defeat NAFLD in their lives.

- *Jim Lowrance*

About the Author:

I am a husband, father, grandfather and lifetime contract salesman, with experience in health writing that began in 2004. I completed theological studies with Liberty University in 1996. I formerly served as editor and forum moderator of Thyroid Health for a major multi-topic content site and as a general health writer for another, where I achieved Editor's Choice Awards for my articles on health subjects.

In 2003 I was diagnosed with hypothyroidism; "Hashimoto's thyroiditis" being the cause. This autoimmune form of thyroid disease that causes destruction of the thyroid gland resulted in my also developing "Chronic Fatigue Syndrome", due to a compromised immune system with severe co-morbid "Adrenal Fatigue".

I also suffered severe anxiety symptoms, including panic attacks early into the onset of Hashimoto's thyroiditis (Hashitoxicosis).

A common, benign heart murmur I was diagnosed with in my teens called "Mitral Valve Prolapse", also worsened in severity of symptoms, with the development of these other health disorders.

My eventual receiving of diagnoses was a difficult process with proper diagnostic testing not being ordered by the first doctors I sought treatment from. These types of issues were inspiration for me to become proactive in my own health care and to self-educate myself on these health disorders, which I have done extensively since 2003.

I now enjoy sharing this information with other patients experiencing my same health disorders.

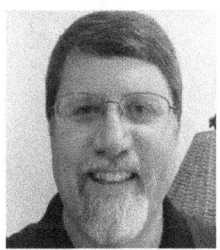

Very Common NonAlcoholic Fatty Liver Disease